Being Rosie

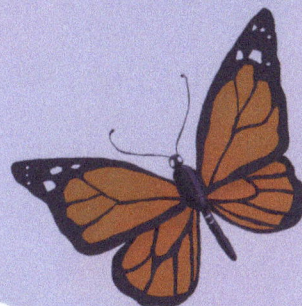

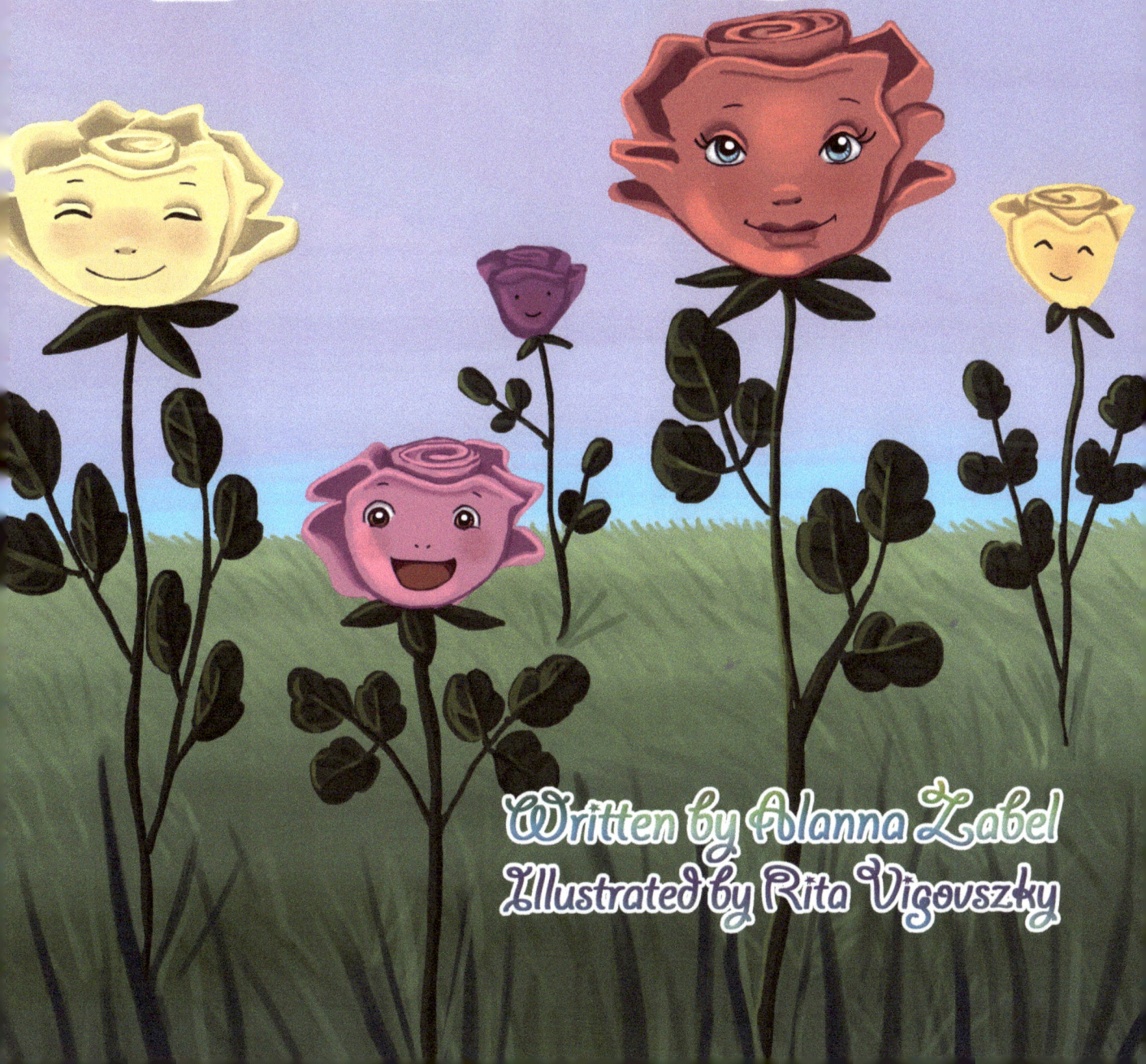

Written by Alanna Zabel

Illustrated by Rita Vigovszky

Published by AZIAM Books.
© 2004, Alanna Zabel.

ISBN-13: 978-0-986-2075-3-2

AZIAM Books
Santa Monica, CA
www.aziam.com

AZ[]AM
BOOKS

Out in the garden
Grew a million wild flowers
Weathering all of the seasons
Sun, snow, and rain showers.

One bud stood above
She was alone of her kind
A beautiful red rose
Hoping a partner to find.

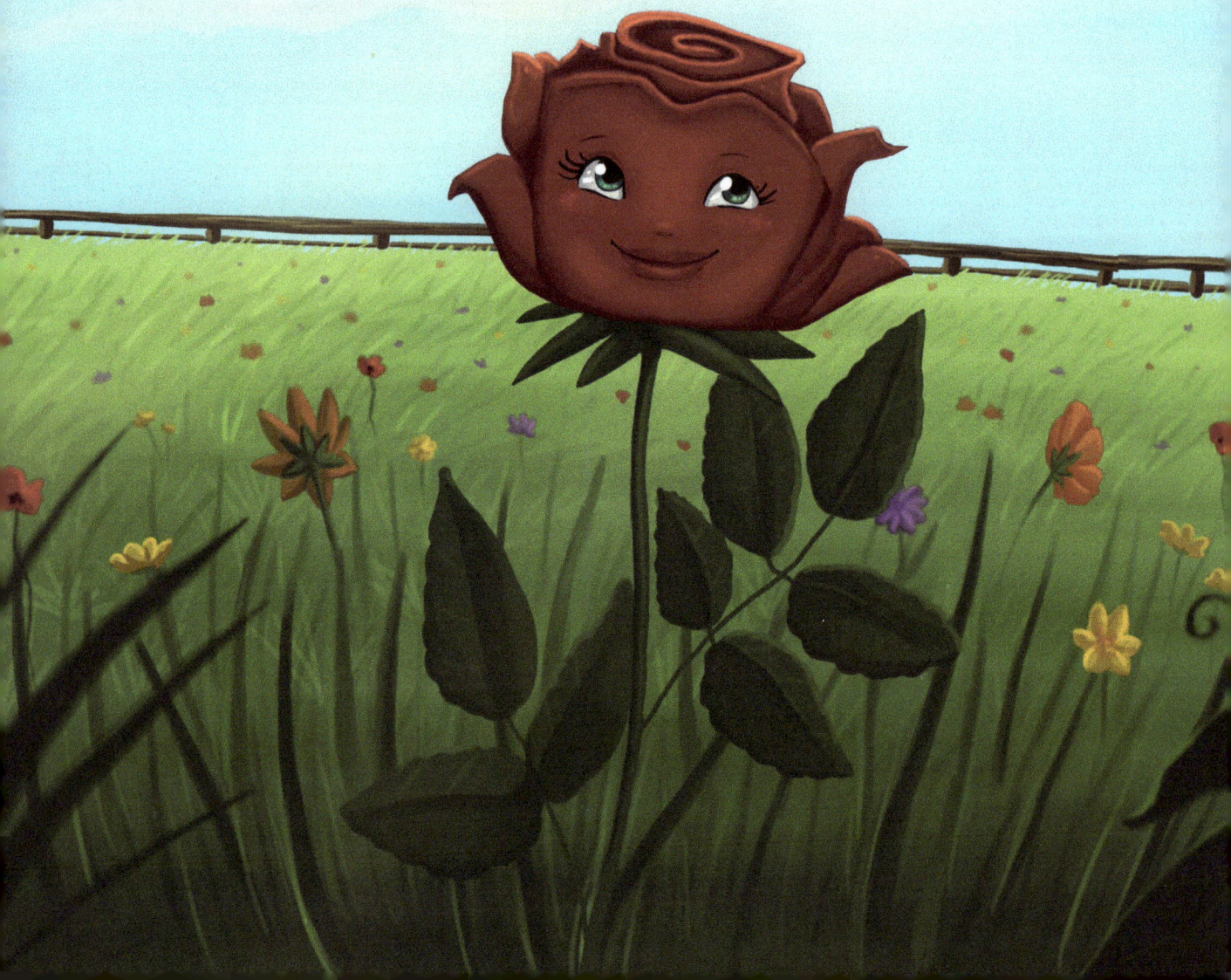

Jealous of her beauty
Other flowers made fun
Calling her vain and elite
That she hogged too much sun.

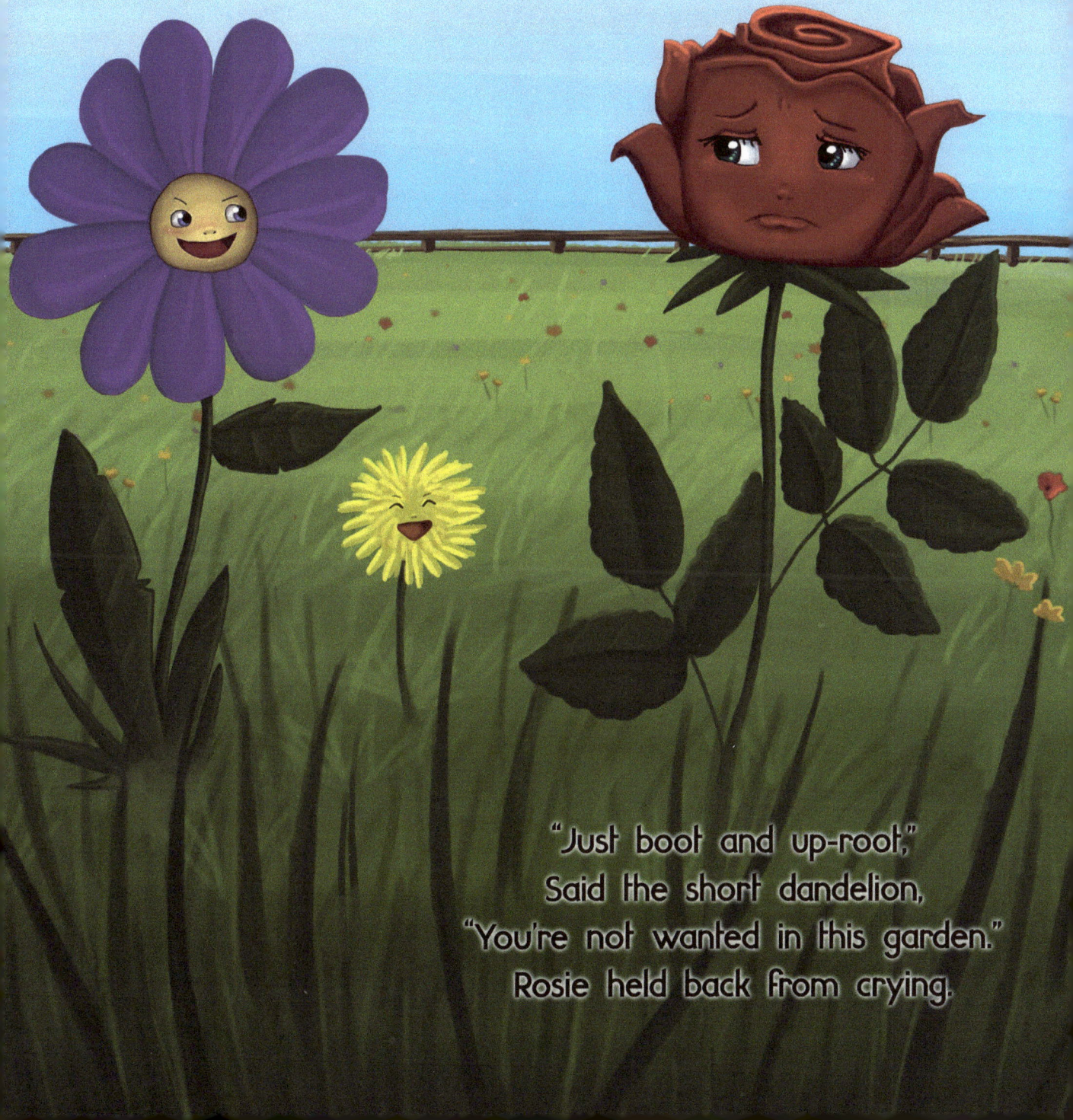

"Just boot and up-root,"
Said the short dandelion,
"You're not wanted in this garden."
Rosie held back from crying.

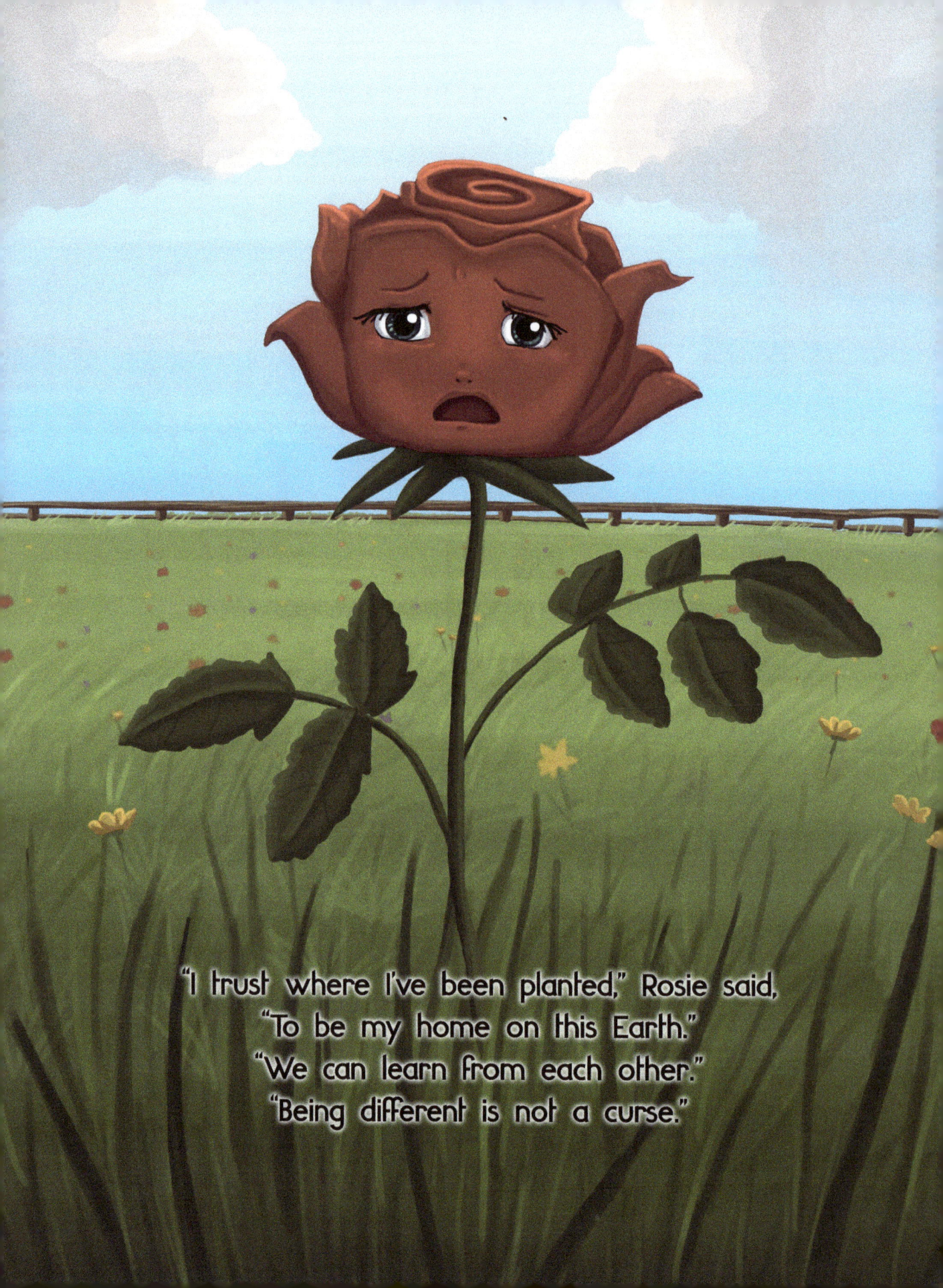

"I trust where I've been planted," Rosie said,
"To be my home on this Earth."
"We can learn from each other."
"Being different is not a curse."

Grass said, "You have thorns on your stem,"
"So animals don't bite."
"I've seen my family eaten,"
"While you bask in the sunlight."

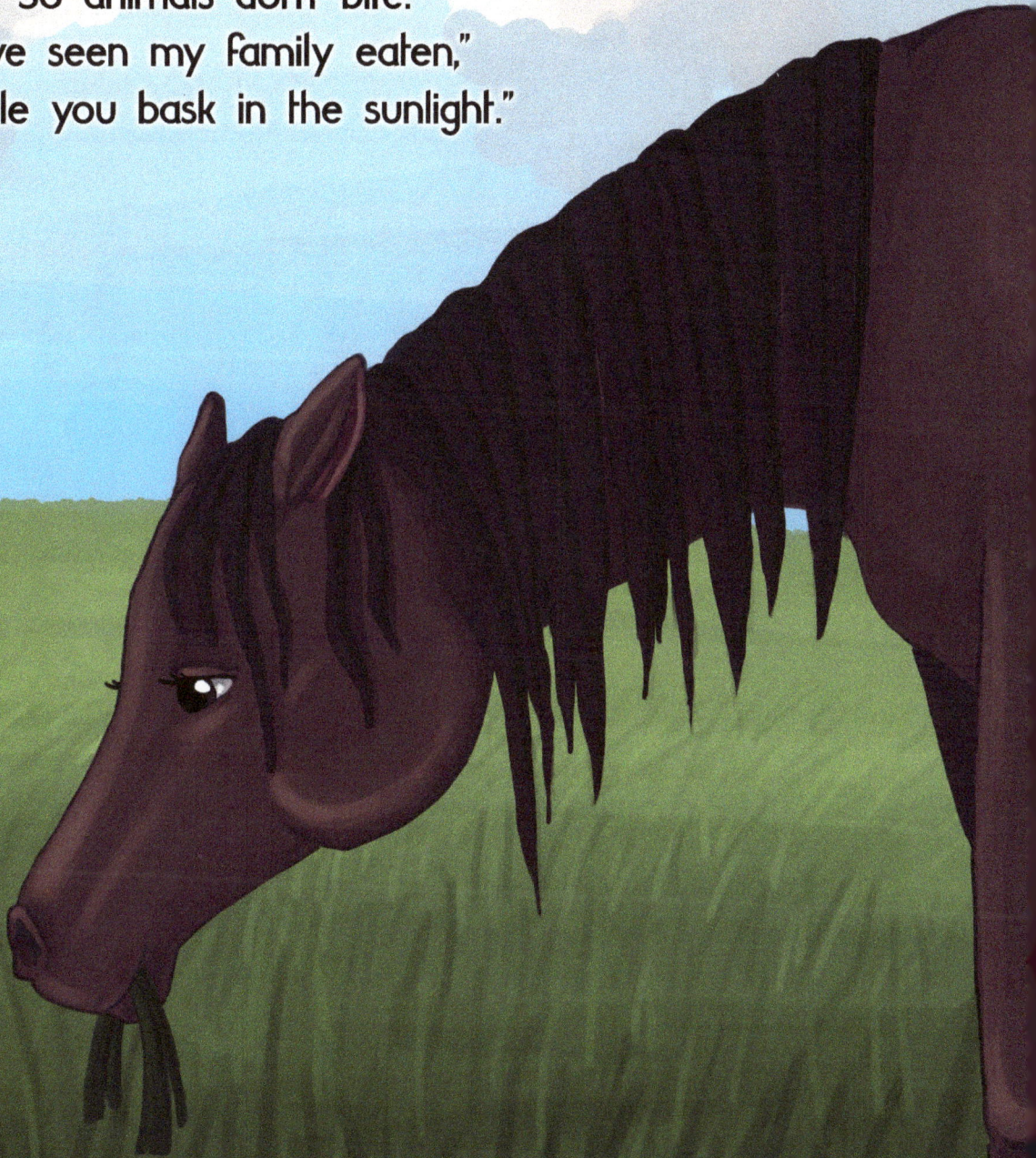

"It's not my fault," Rosie said,
"I am what I am."
"You wanting to be me,"
"Creates an identity jam."

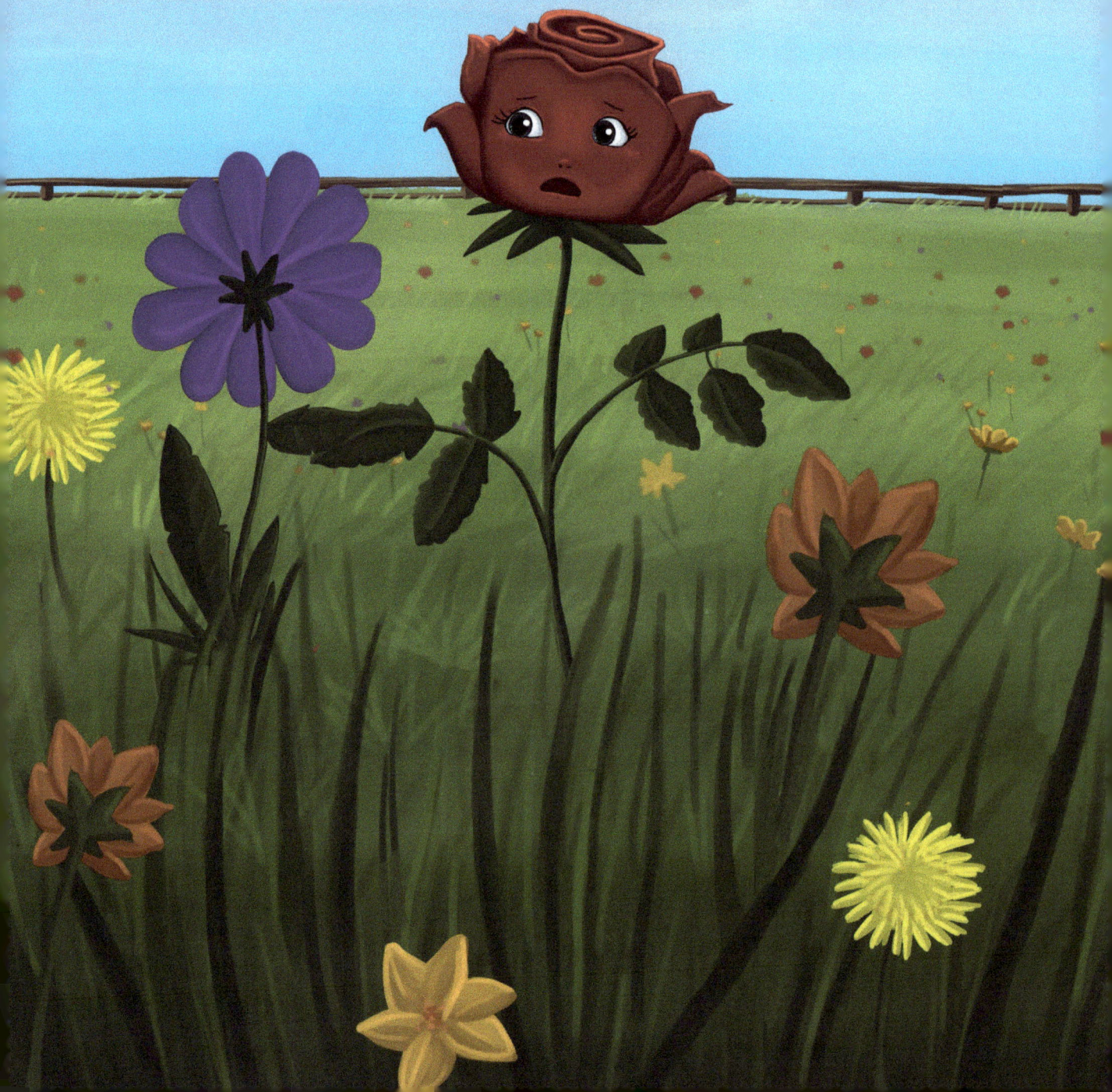

They all laughed in her face
"Rosie, where are you from?"
"No one cares what you think,"
"And what you think is dumb."

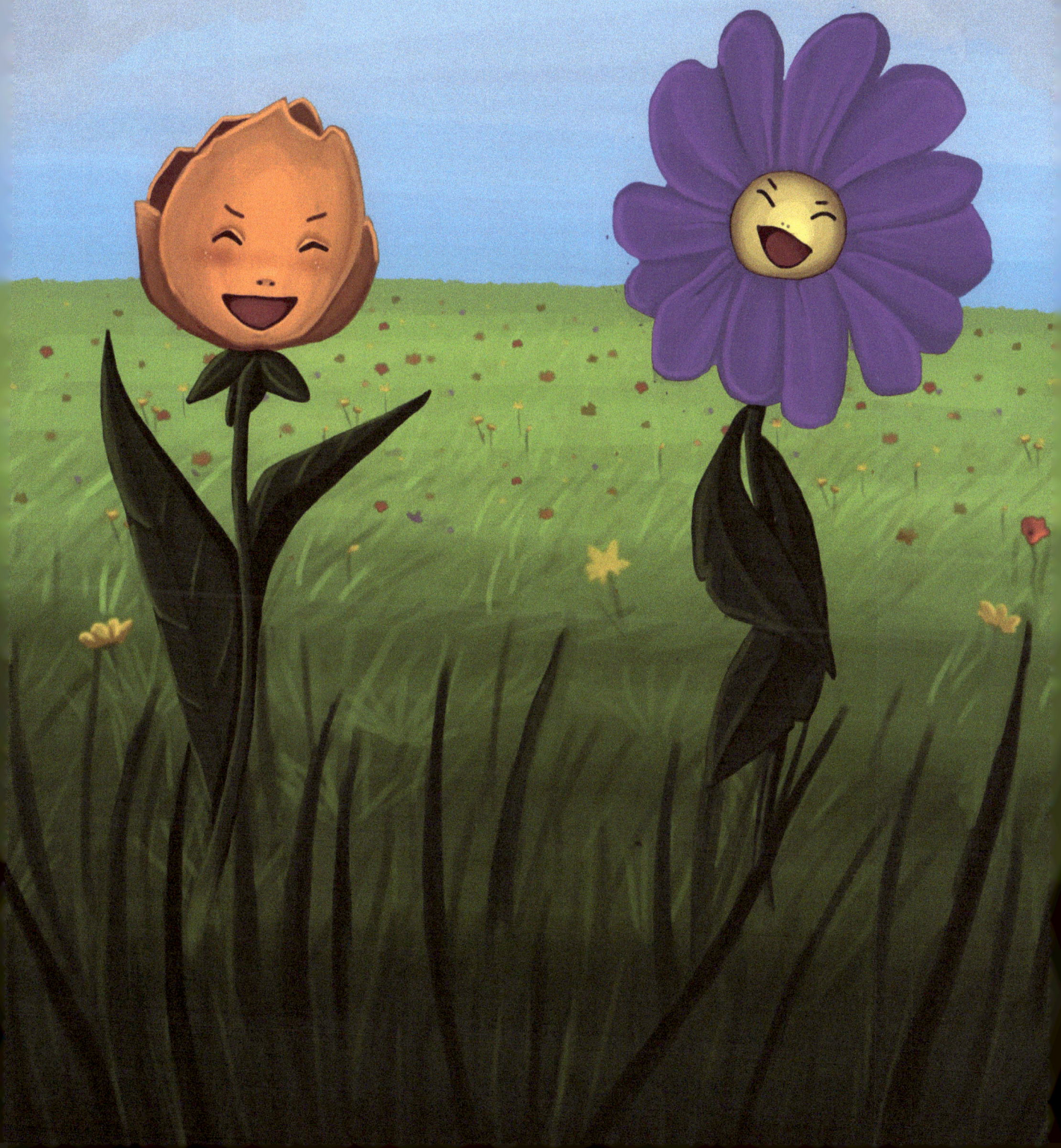

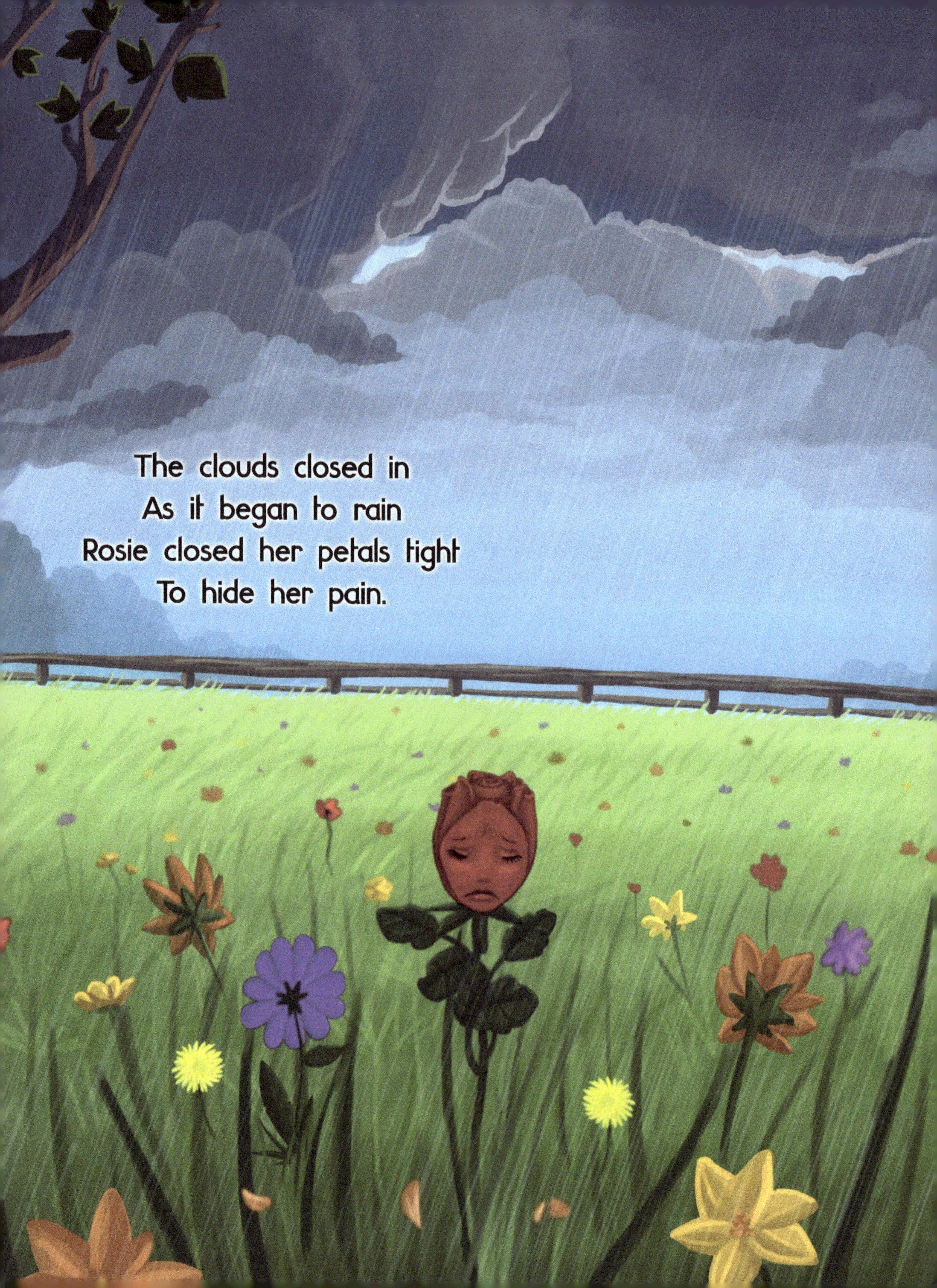

The clouds closed in
As it began to rain
Rosie closed her petals tight
To hide her pain.

The plants rejoiced the next morning
When the Sun presented the day.
They soaked in the energy
From each solar ray.

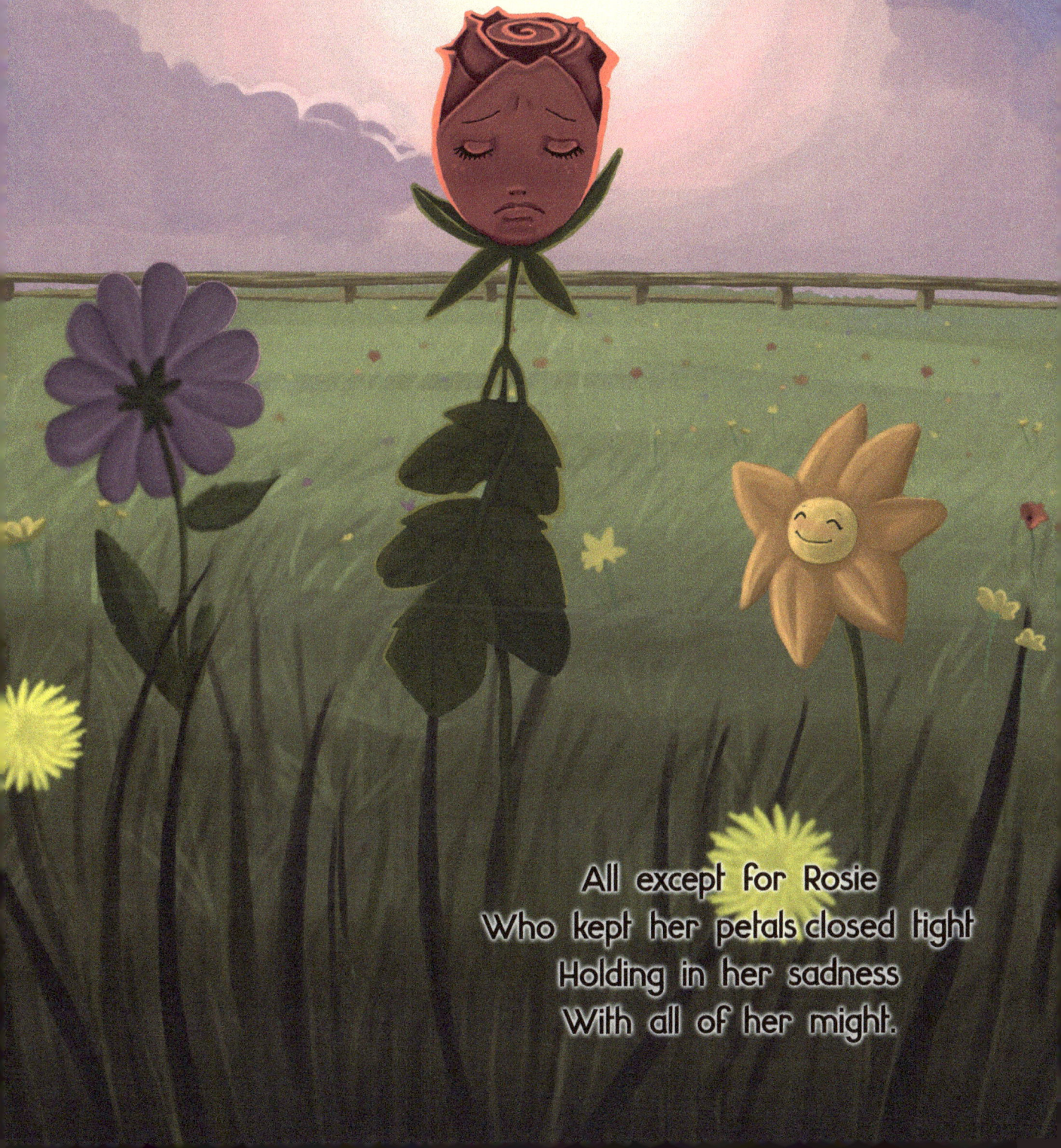

All except for Rosie
Who kept her petals closed tight
Holding in her sadness
With all of her might.

Buzzy Bumble Bee buzzed by
Pollinating his friends
"What's up with Rosie?" he asked.
"She's pouting," Sprig said.

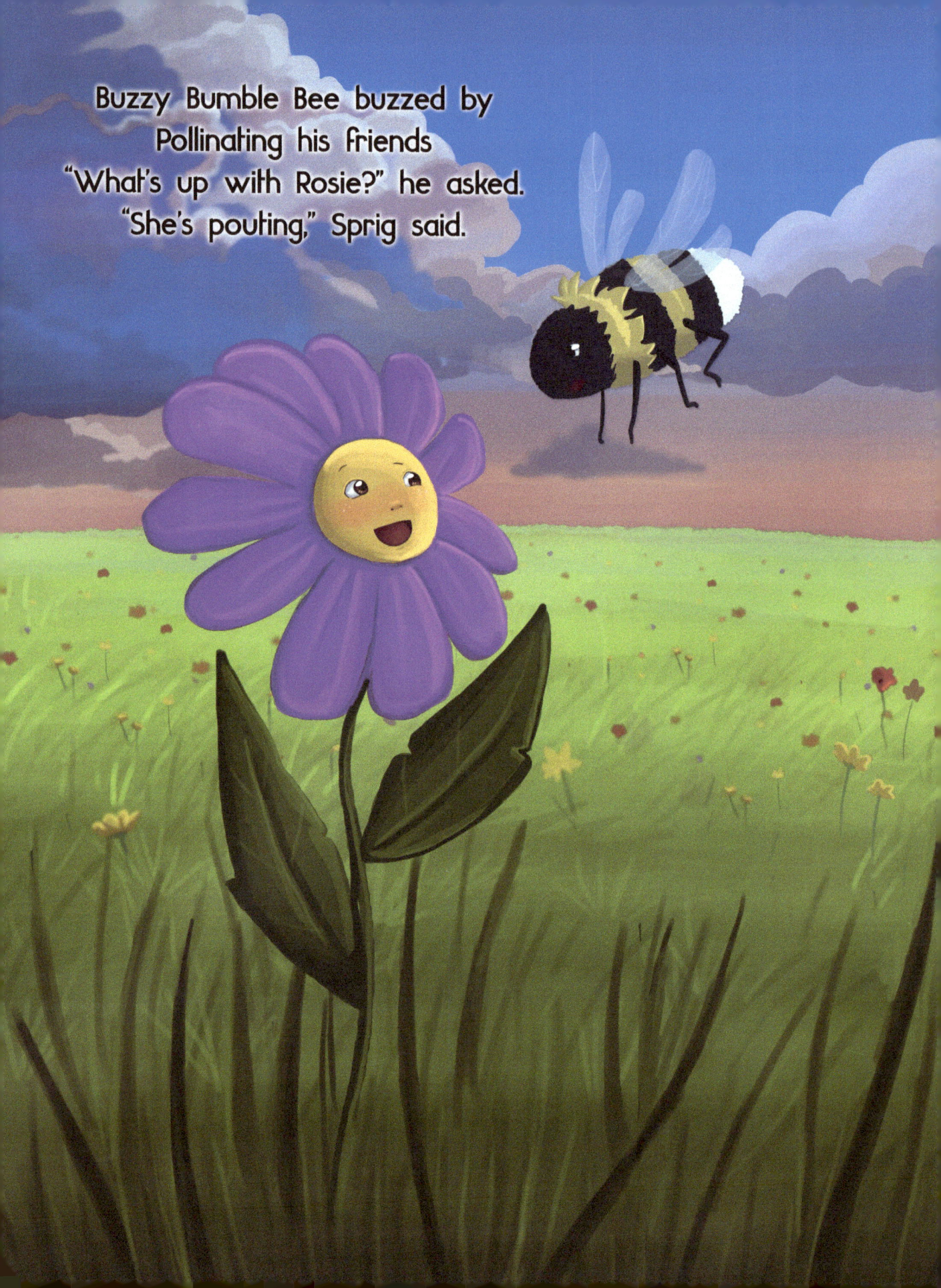

Rosie's stem began to droop
Her color had faded
After four days of hiding
She was severely dehydrated.

"She's not drinking any water,"
"Or taking any light,"
"From the looks of her," said Pine Tree
"She won't make it through the night."

"It's not our fault," Grass said,
"She chose to quit"
"She is the one"
"Who felt like a misfit."

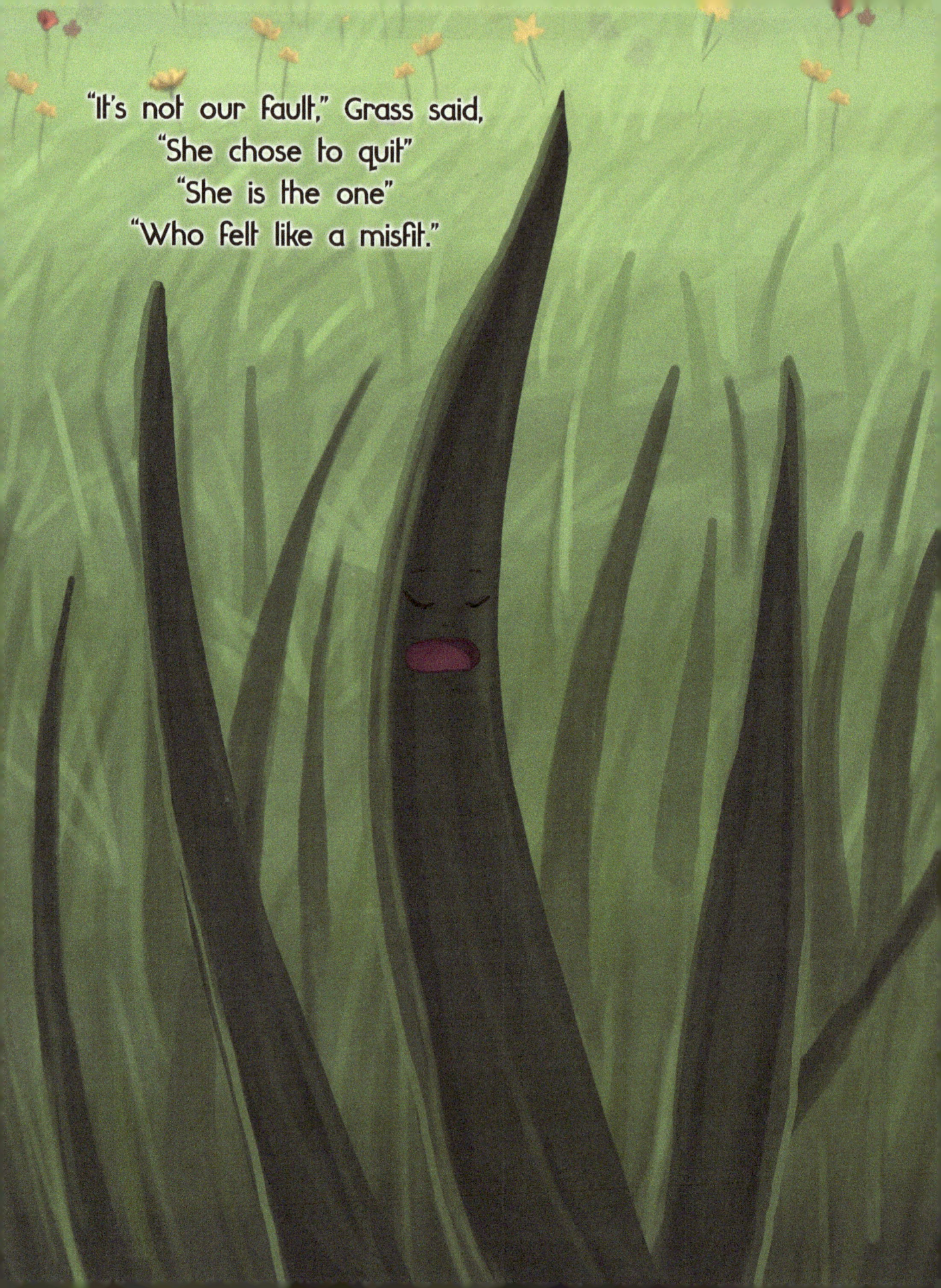

Without any strength left
Rosie breathed out a sigh
She fell to the ground
And appeared to die.

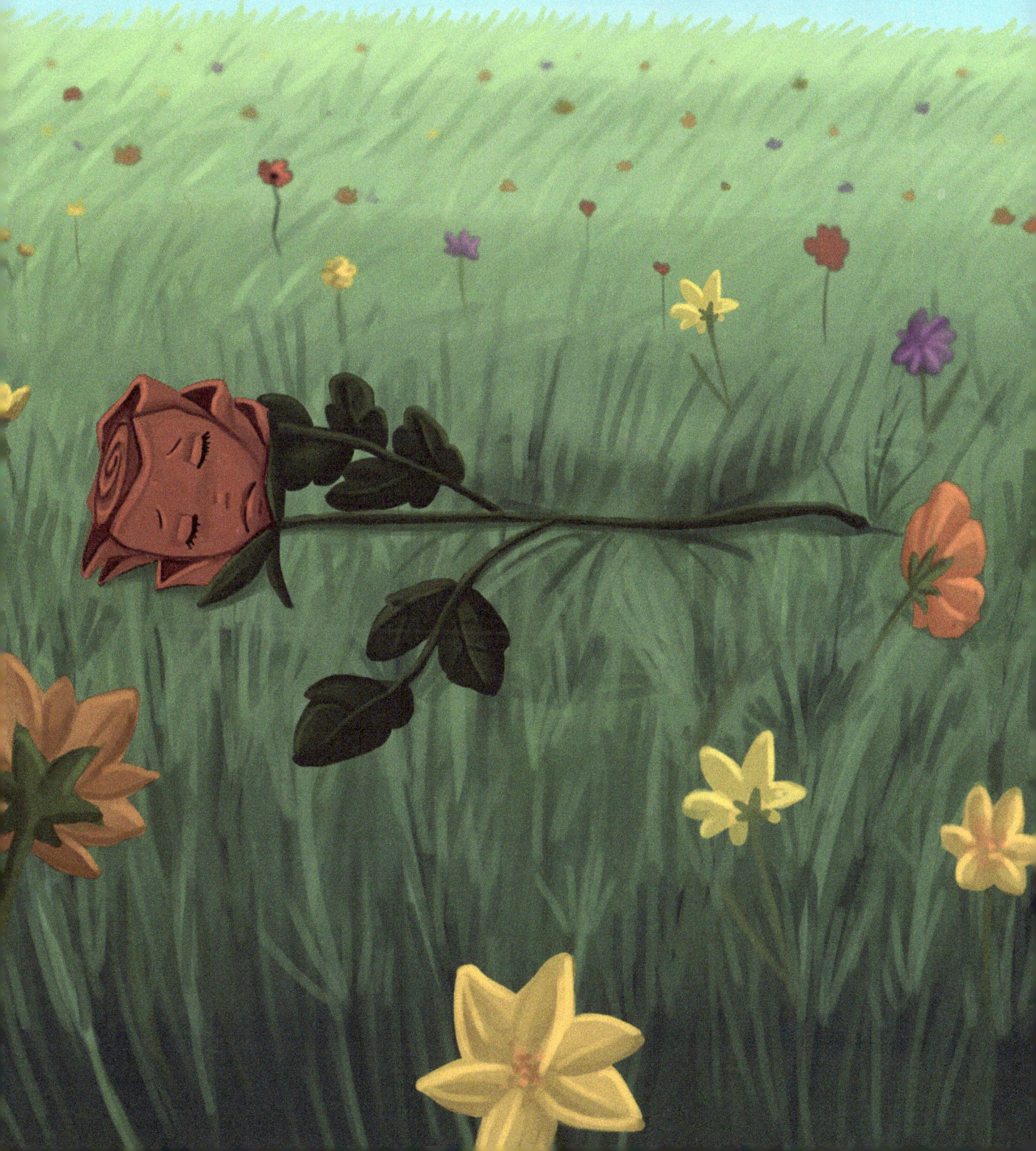

Just then, Farmer walked by
He bent and felt Rosie's leaves
"This rose needs some loving," he said,
"I know just what she needs."

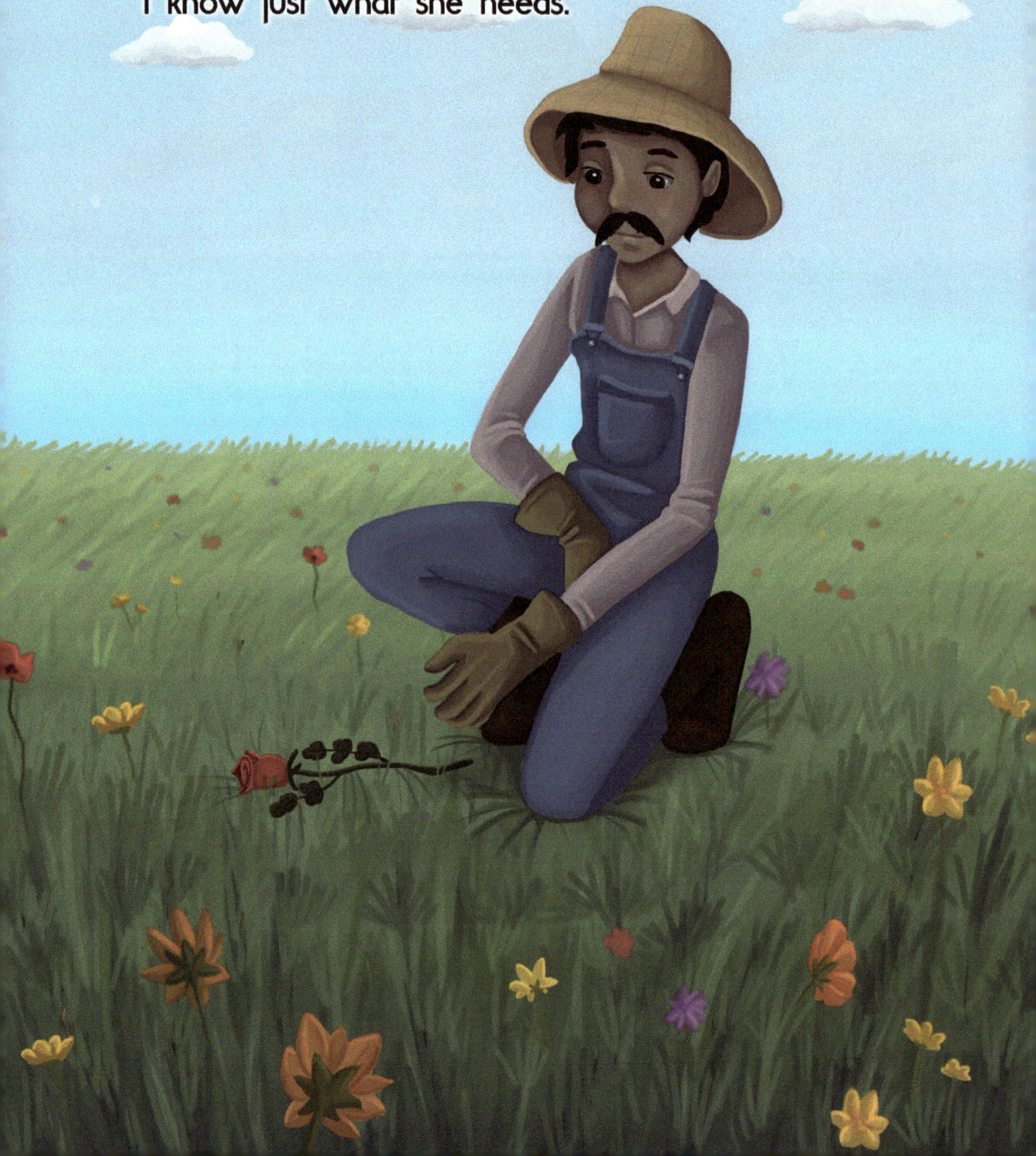

He pulled Rosie from the ground
With no effort at all, it seemed
Then he walked back to his truck
With her roots swinging in the breeze.

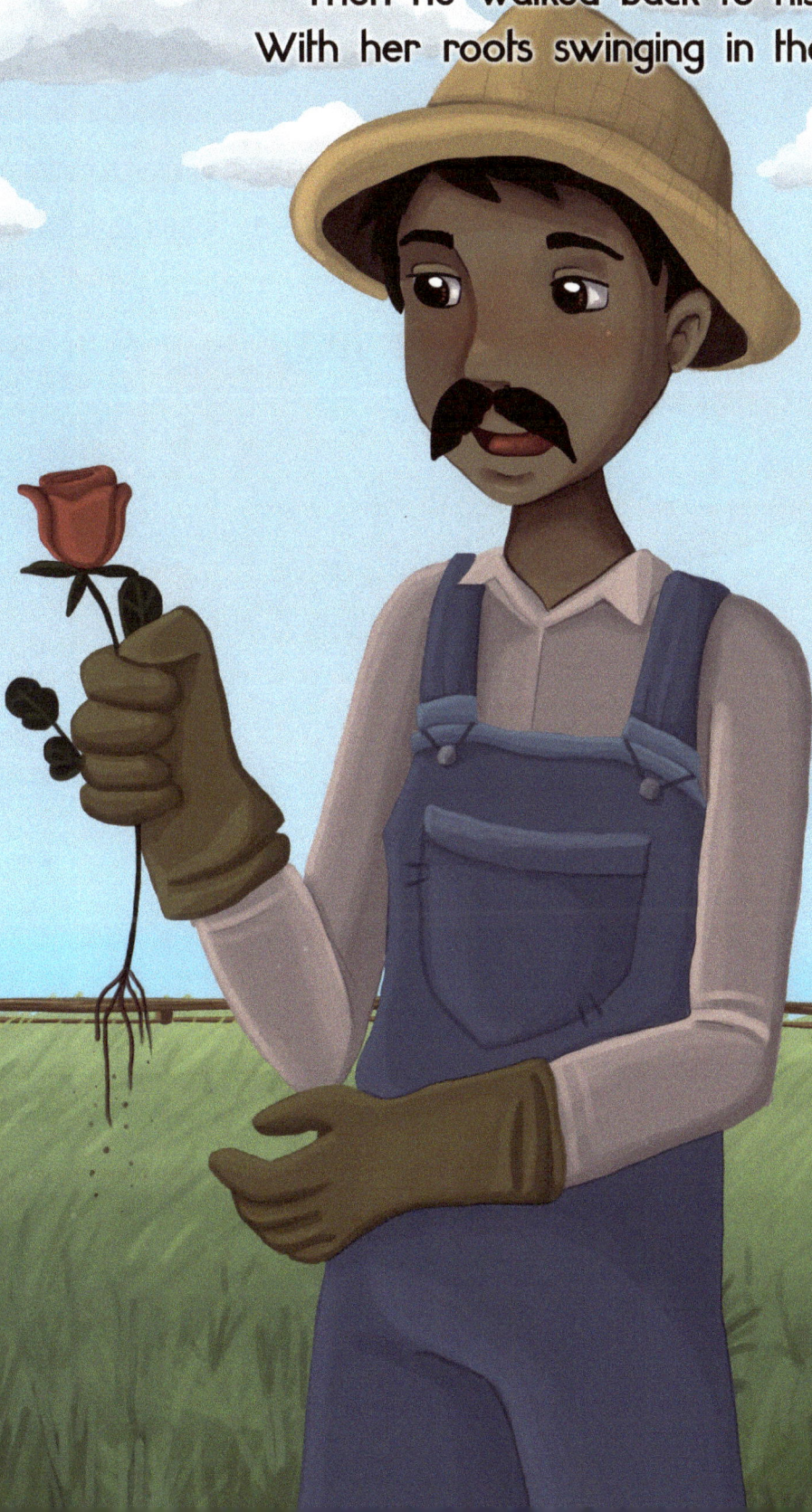

"Hey, wait!" the Garden yelled,
"Who's going to sing?"
"No one else smells as sweet,"
"Or is as inspiring!"

But the Farmer's pick-up drove off
With Rosie tossing about
She was scared and cold
And then she passed out.

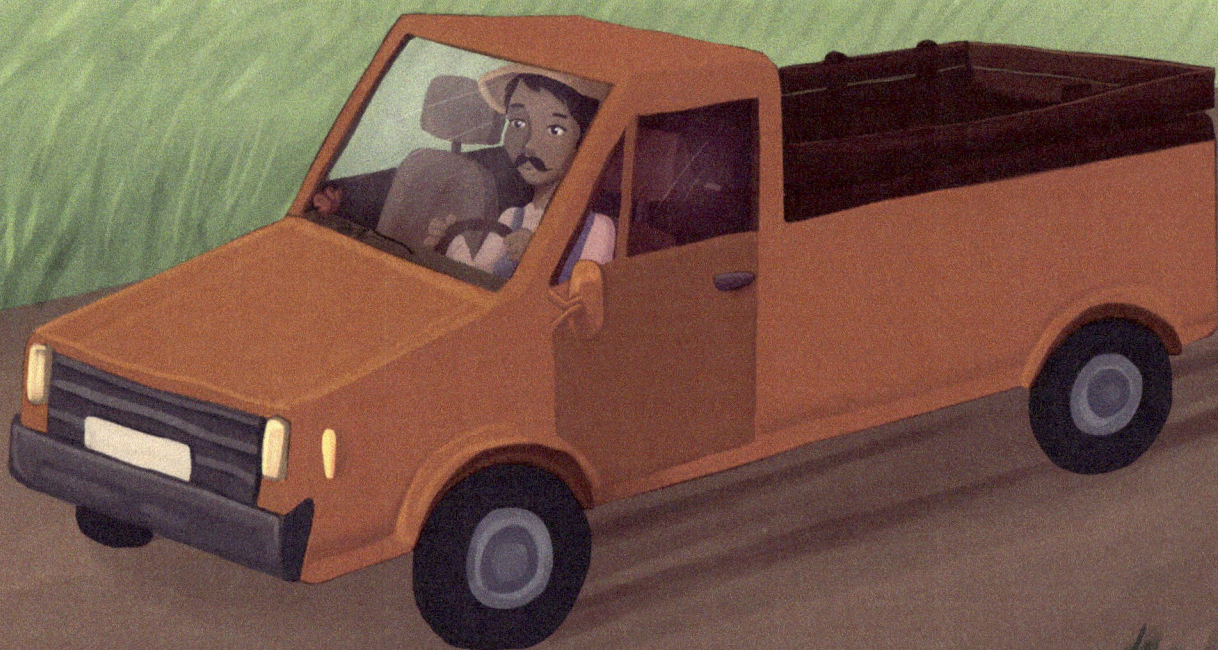

As the Sun rose the next morning
Rosie awoke, too
She smelled the sweetest aroma
The Earth felt warm and new.

She was surrounded with flowers
Who looked just like her
Yellow, blue, white, and purple
This was Heaven for sure.

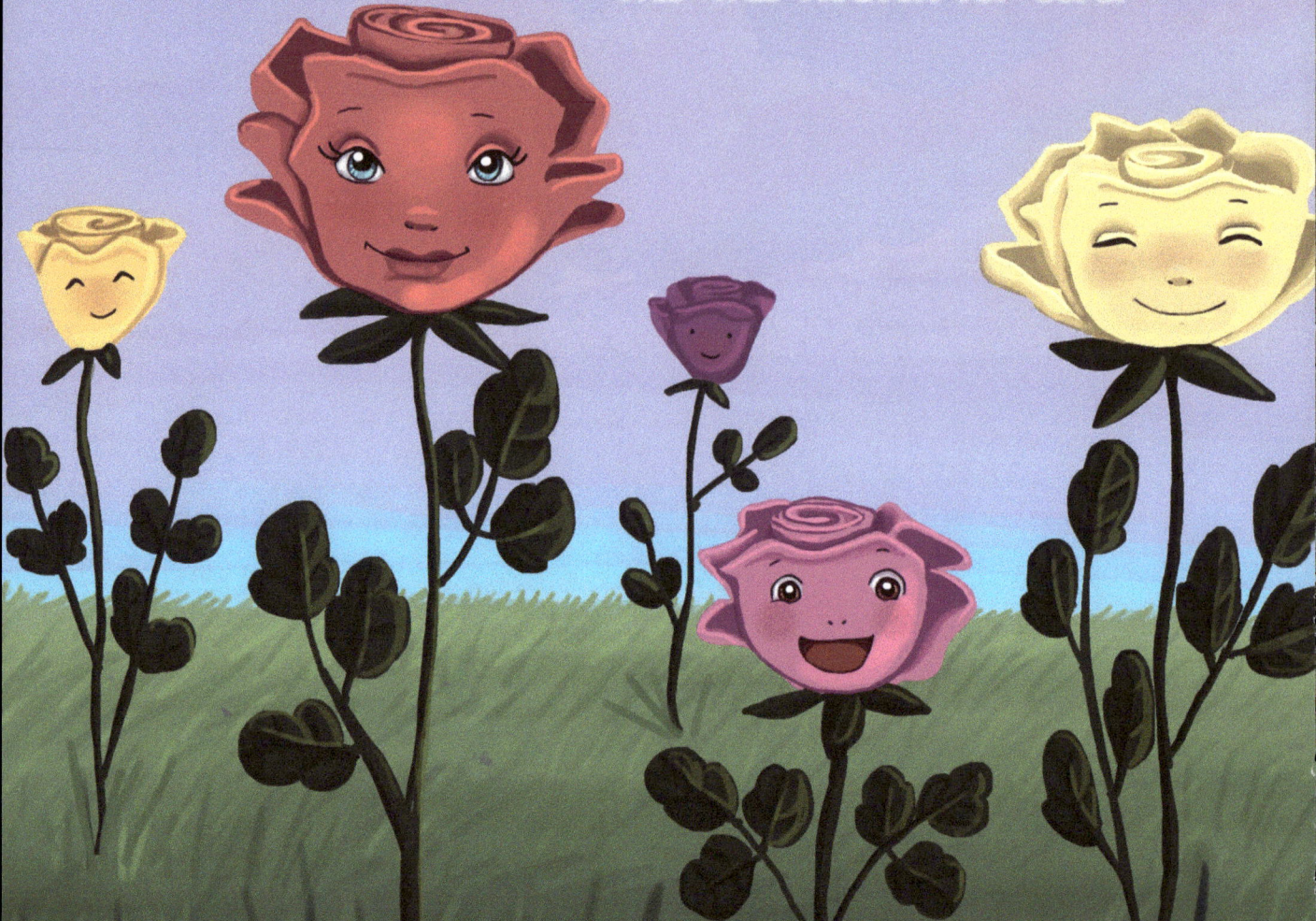

"I'm not alone anymore," she thought
"There's more of my kind"
"But how will they accept me?"
"I'm all dried up," she whined.

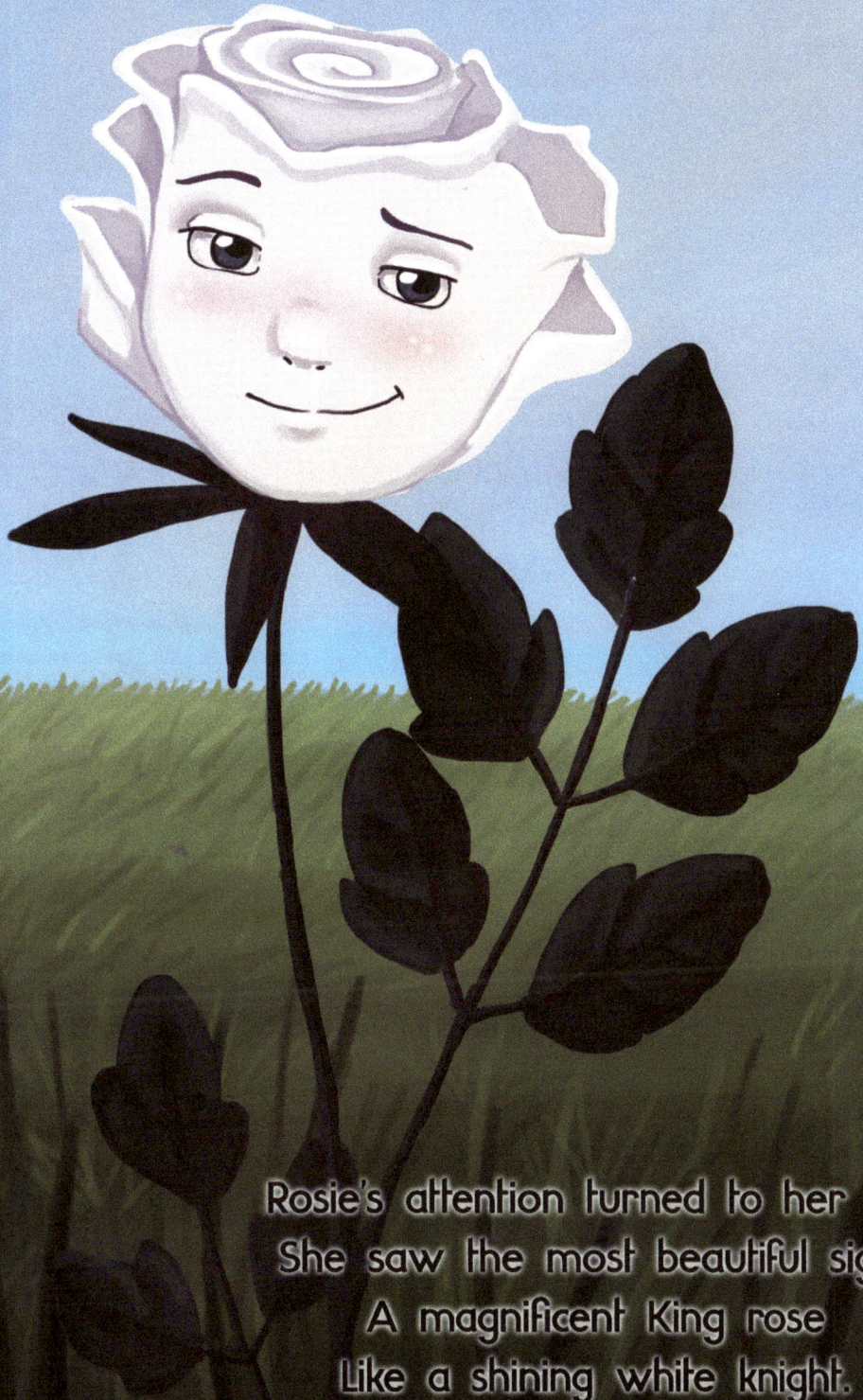

Rosie's attention turned to her left
She saw the most beautiful sight
A magnificent King rose
Like a shining white knight.

"You sing like an angel," he said,
"Your voice is sweet and pure,"
"My name is Bud,"
"You belong here, for sure."

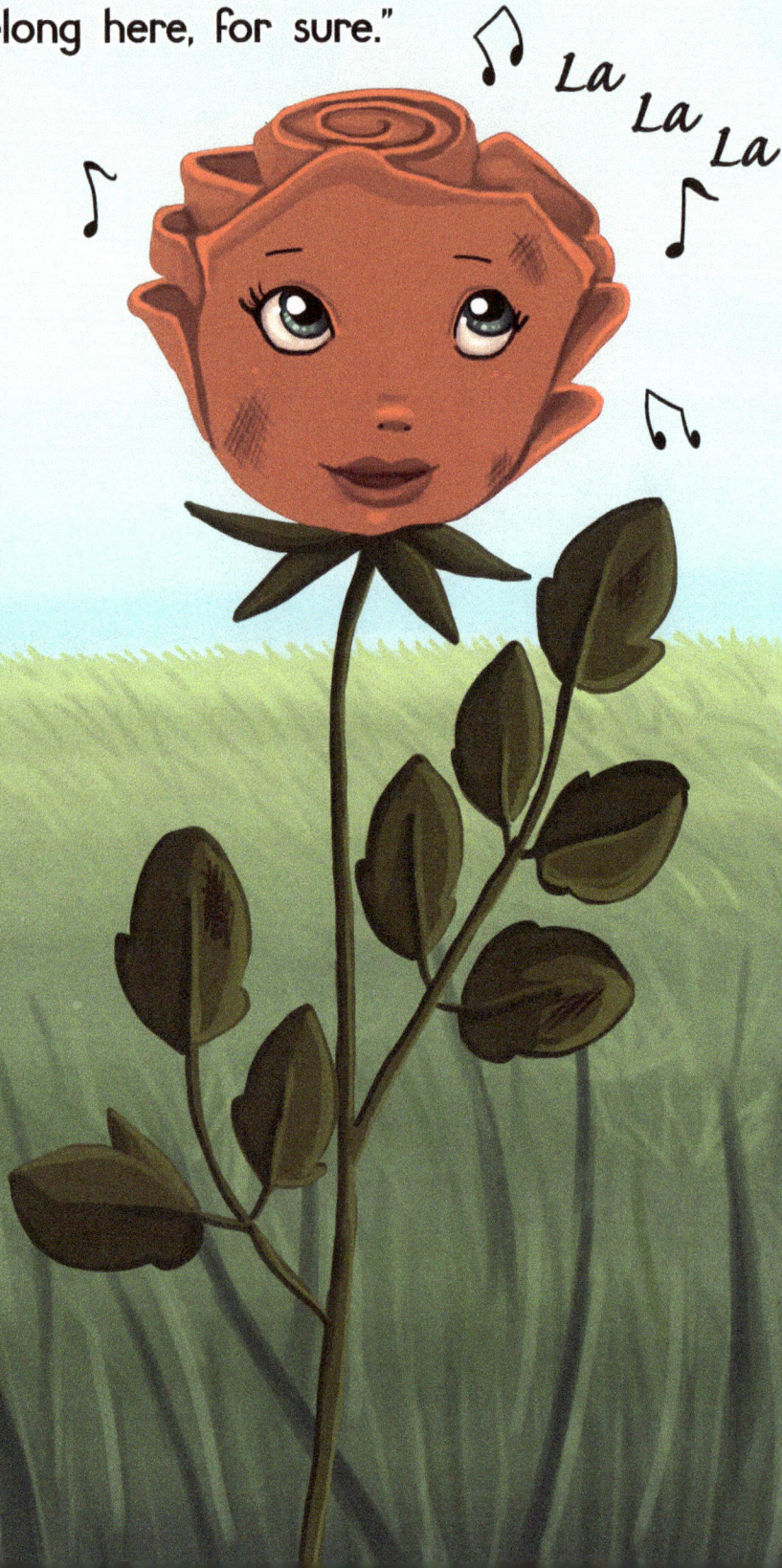

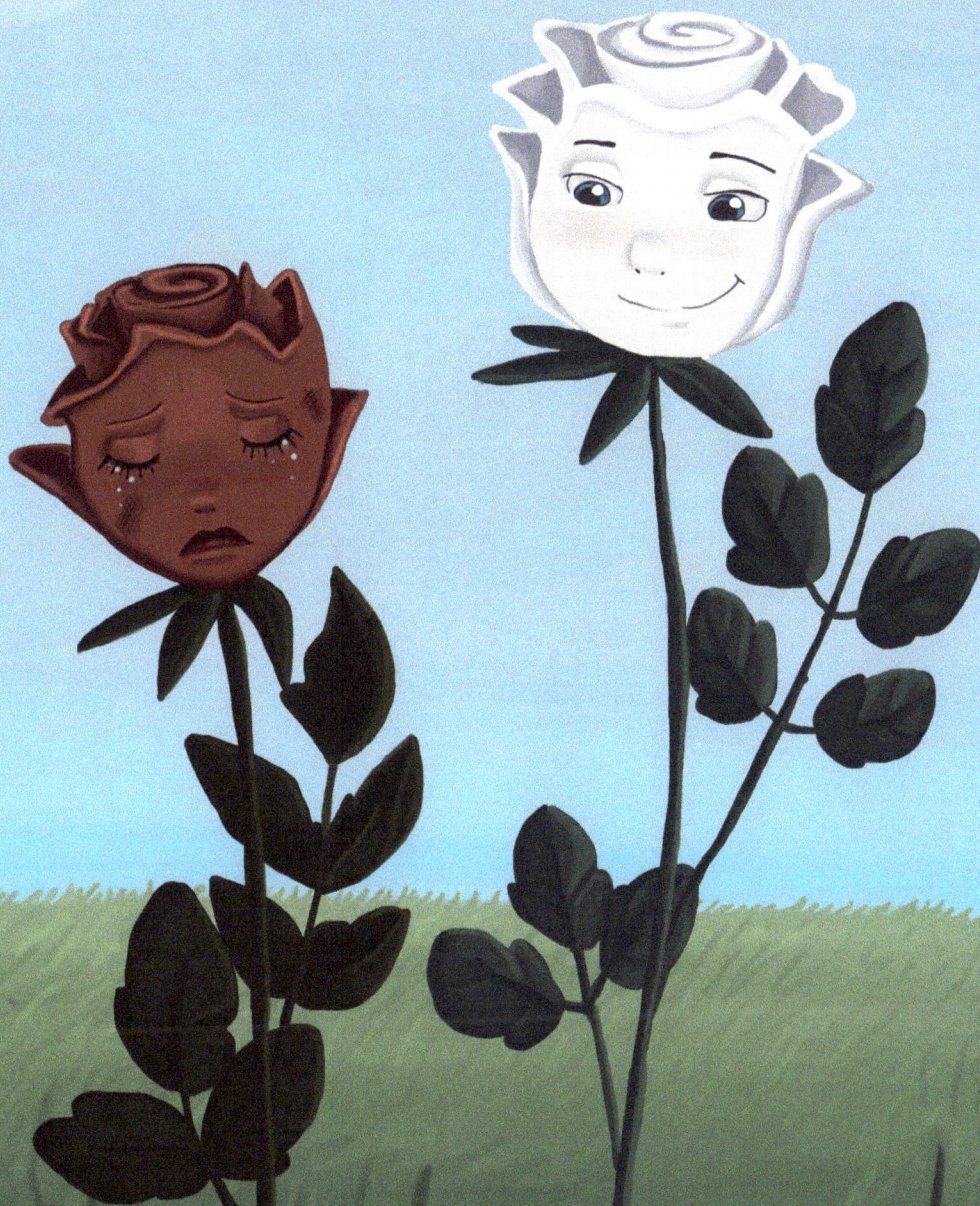

"I've grown three times more thorns," Rosie said,
"My petals are all dried out,"
"I'm scared I'll be laughed at,"
"And I can't help but pout."

"I used to be so beautiful," Rosie said,
"Now I only want to hide."
"Everyone is beautiful," said Bud,
"Especially when you look from the inside."

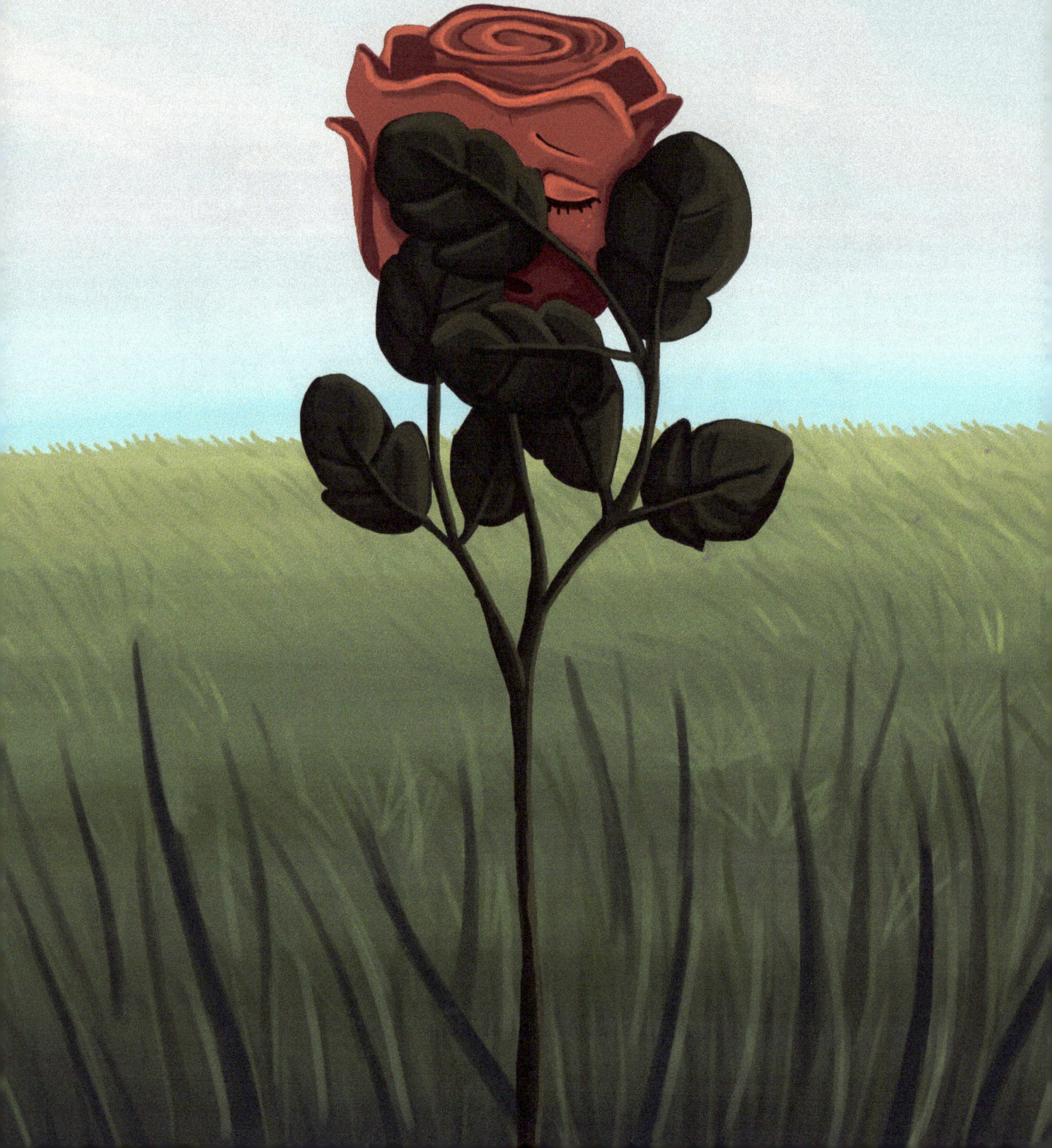

"No one is going to bully you anymore"
"You're with more evolved plants"
"Compassionate, positive, and kind"
"Who love to share, sing, and dance."

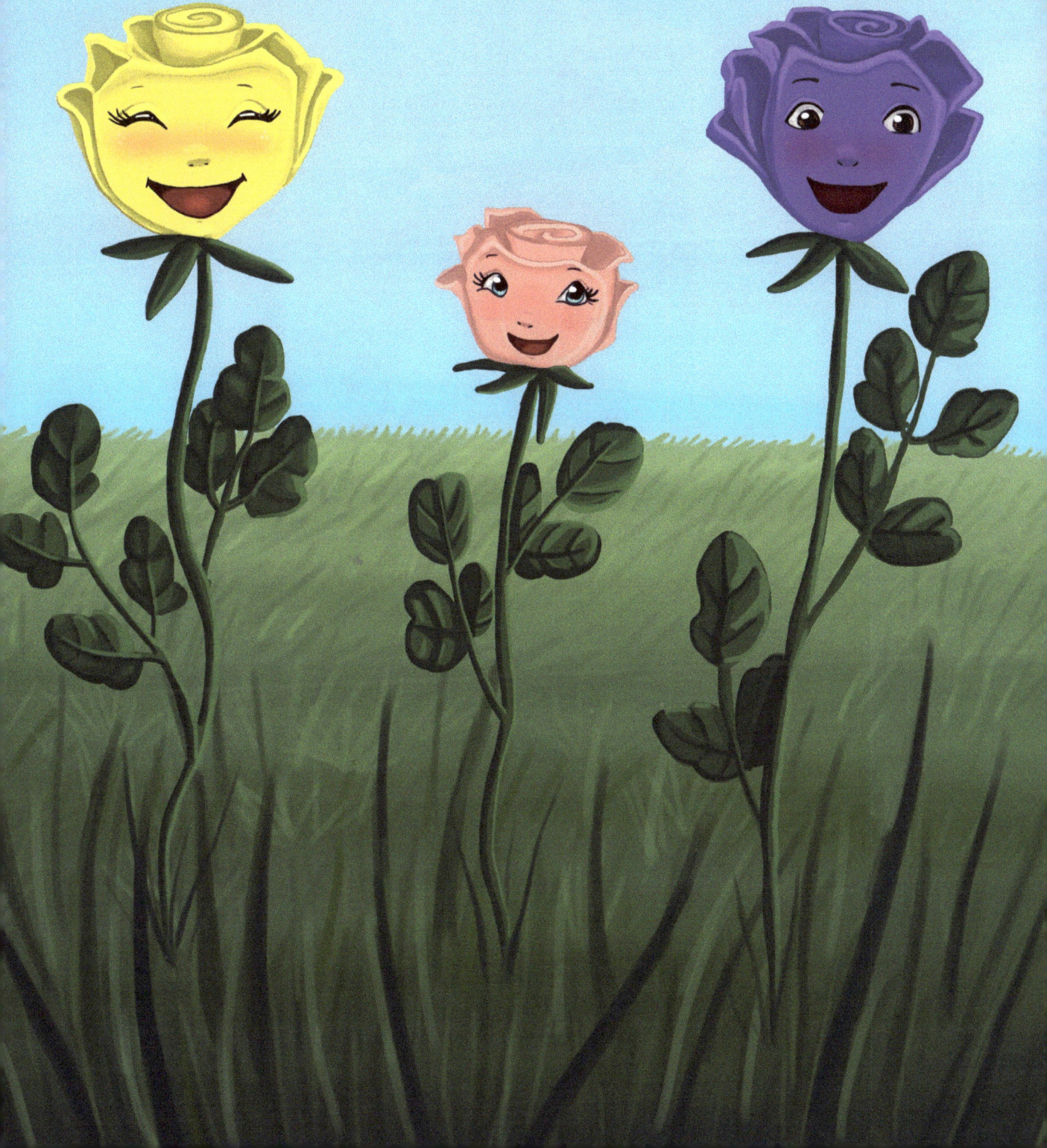

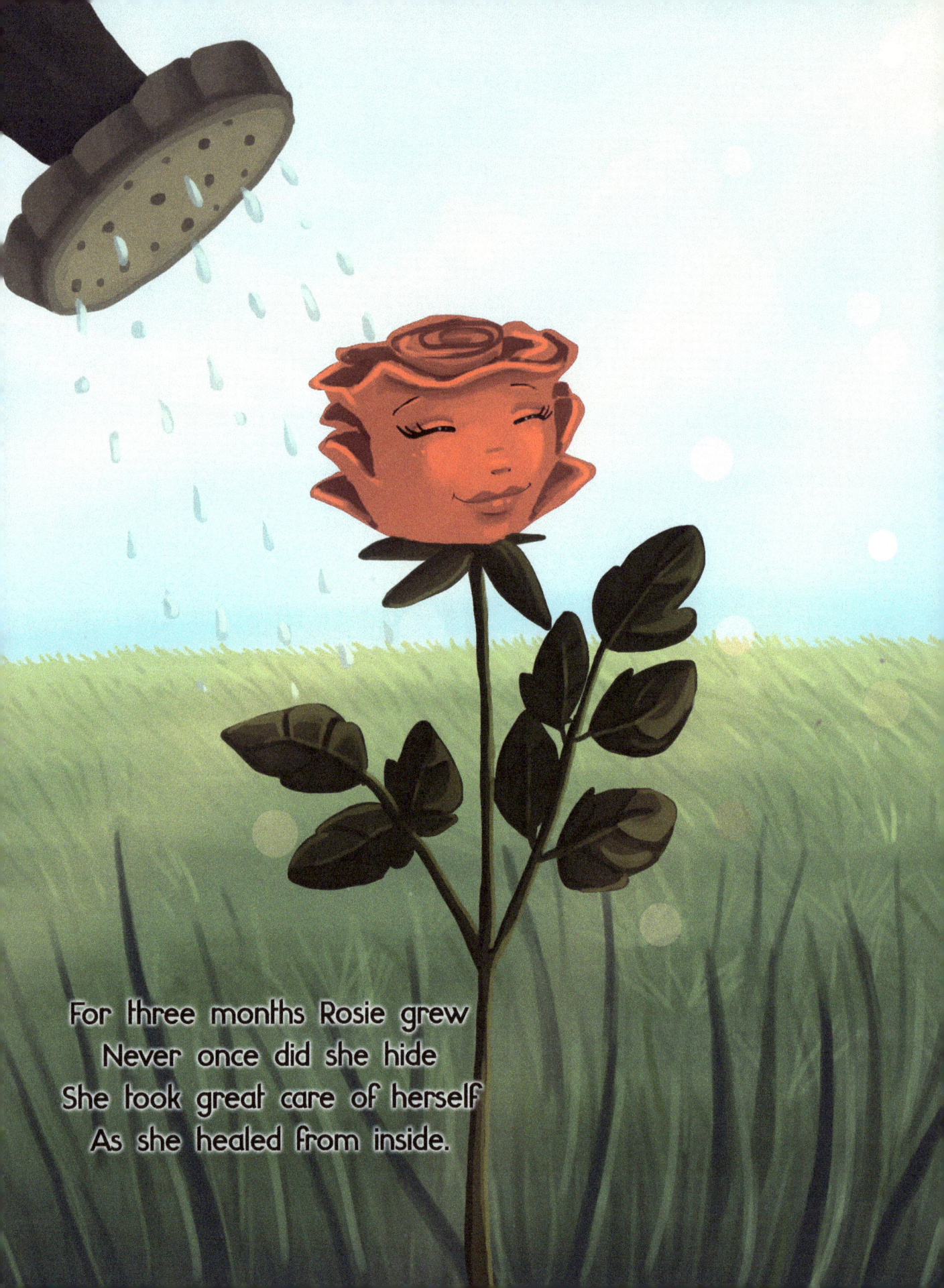

For three months Rosie grew
Never once did she hide
She took great care of herself
As she healed from inside.

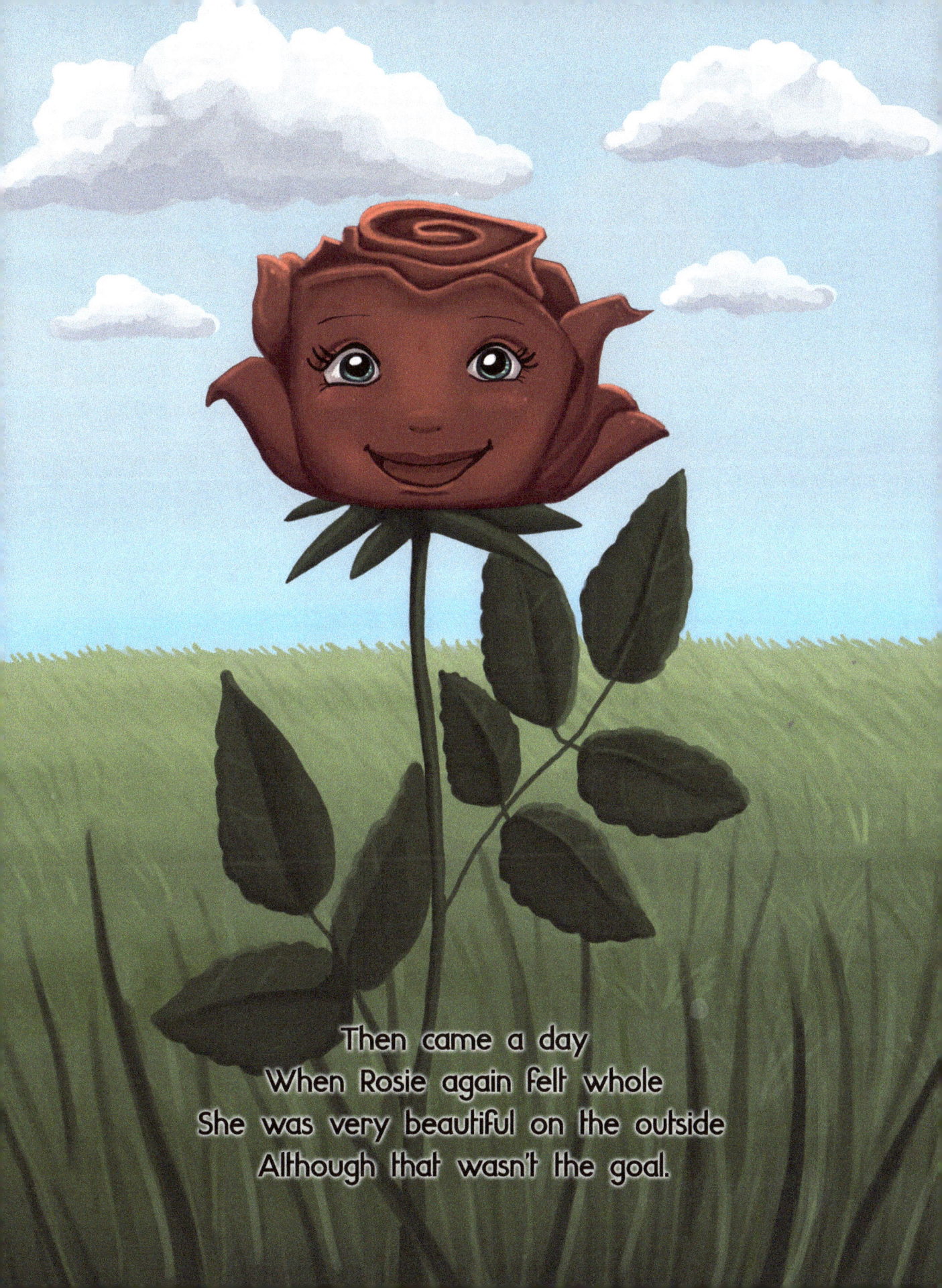

Then came a day
When Rosie again felt whole
She was very beautiful on the outside
Although that wasn't the goal.

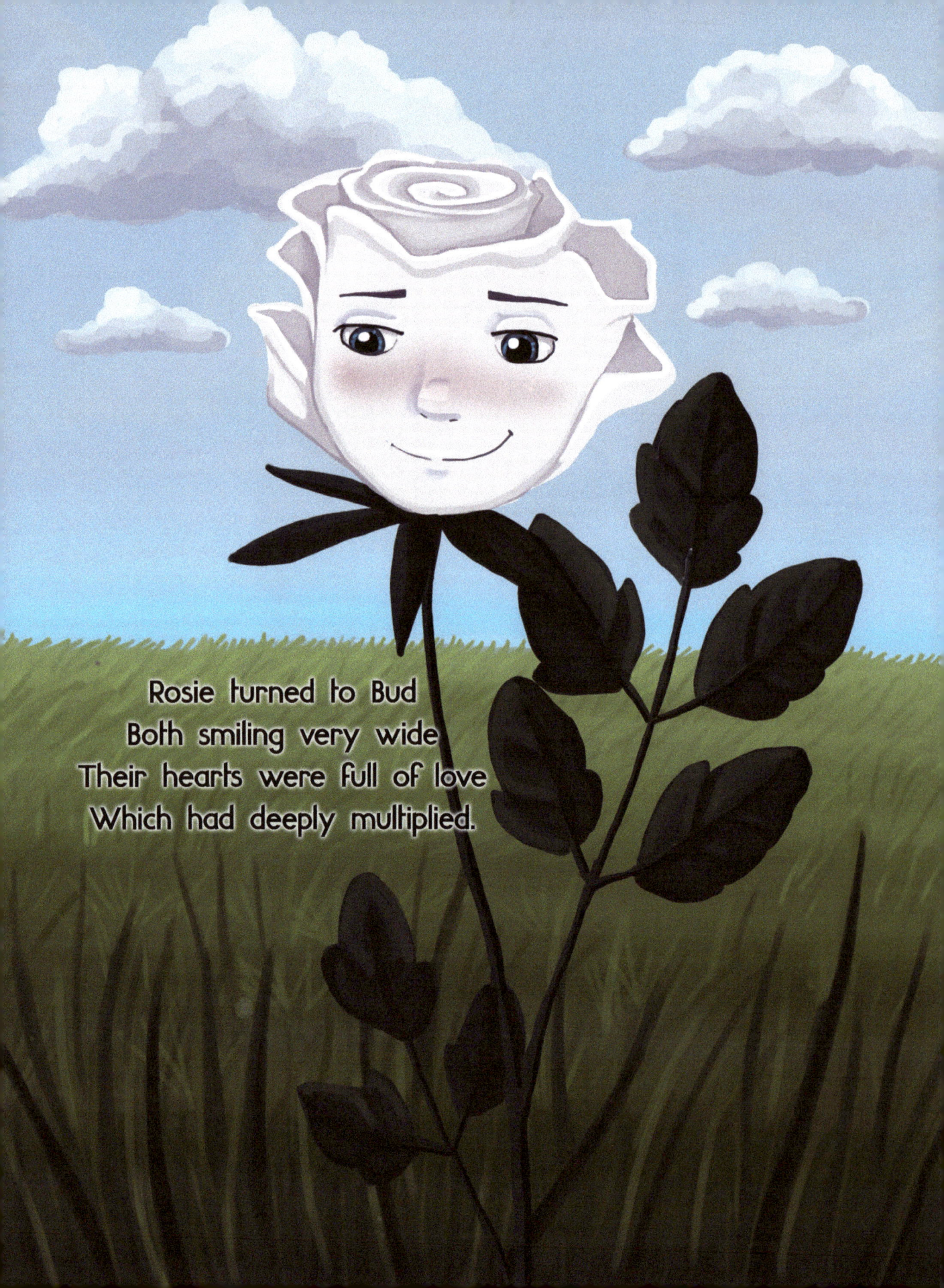

Rosie turned to Bud
Both smiling very wide
Their hearts were full of love
Which had deeply multiplied.

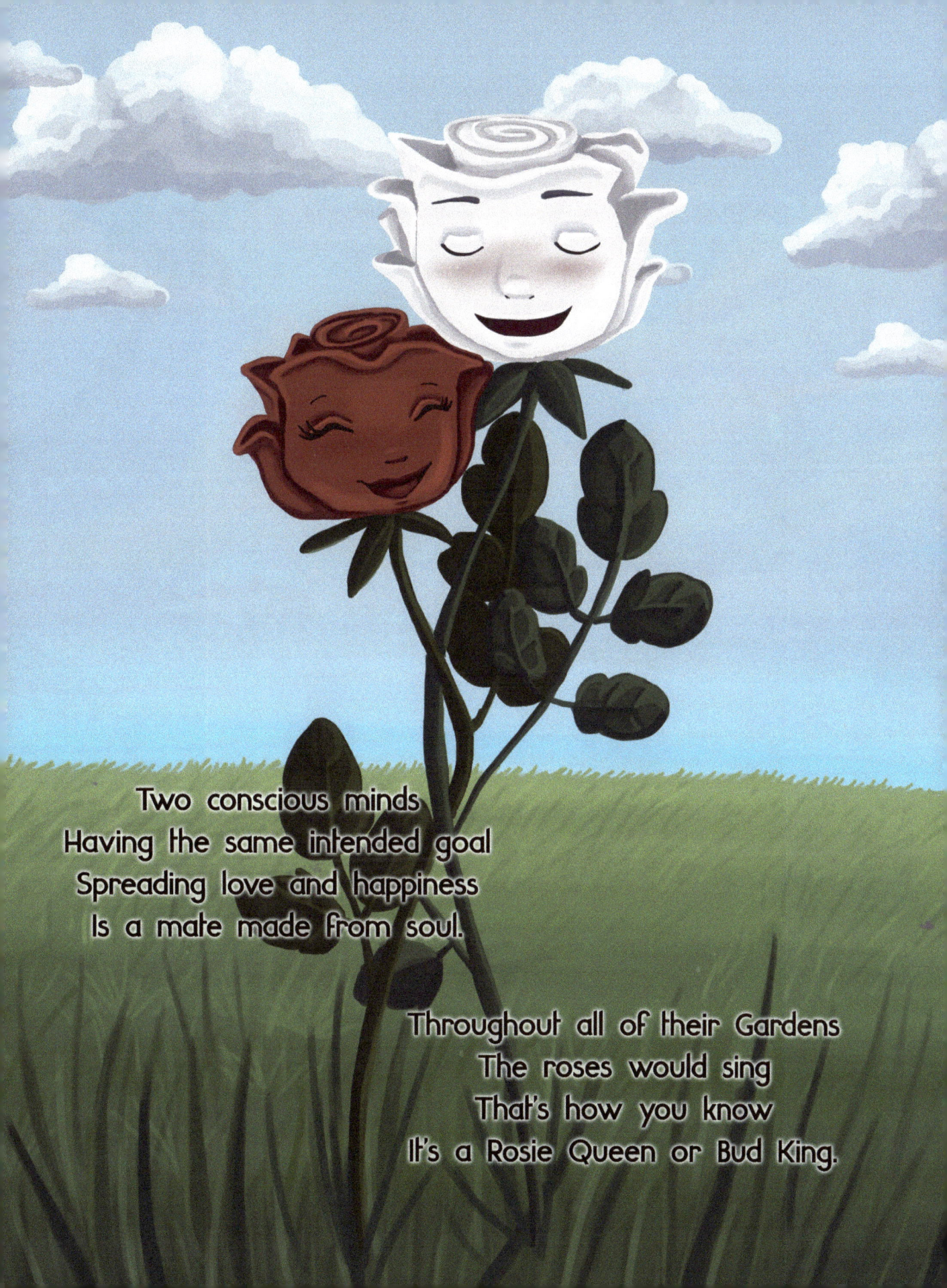

Two conscious minds
Having the same intended goal
Spreading love and happiness
Is a mate made from soul.

Throughout all of their Gardens
The roses would sing
That's how you know
It's a Rosie Queen or Bud King.

Gradually both of the Gardens
Grew closer together
Roses, grass, and dandelions
Enduring all seasons and weather.

Everyone learned to love themselves
For their own unique traits
This led them to love each other
And accept their individual fates.

What is Red? What is Blue?
What is Big or Small?
Wings, feet, or petals
Let's welcome them all!

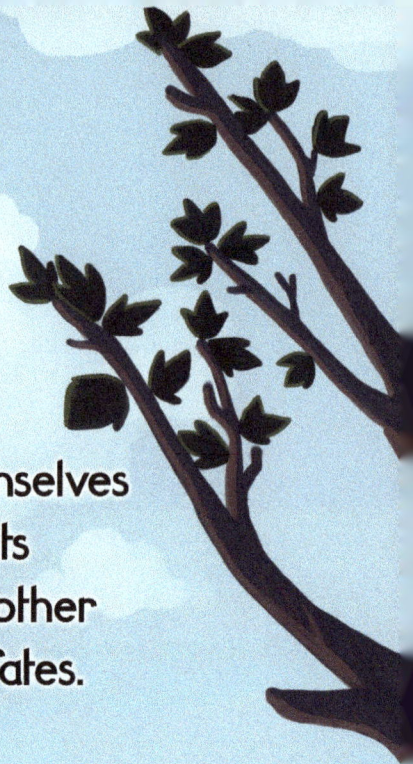

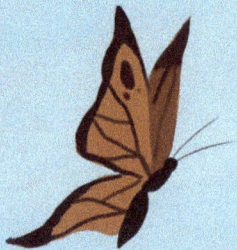

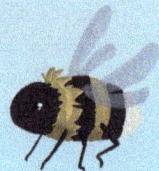

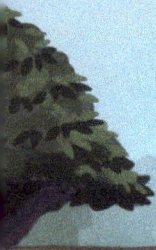

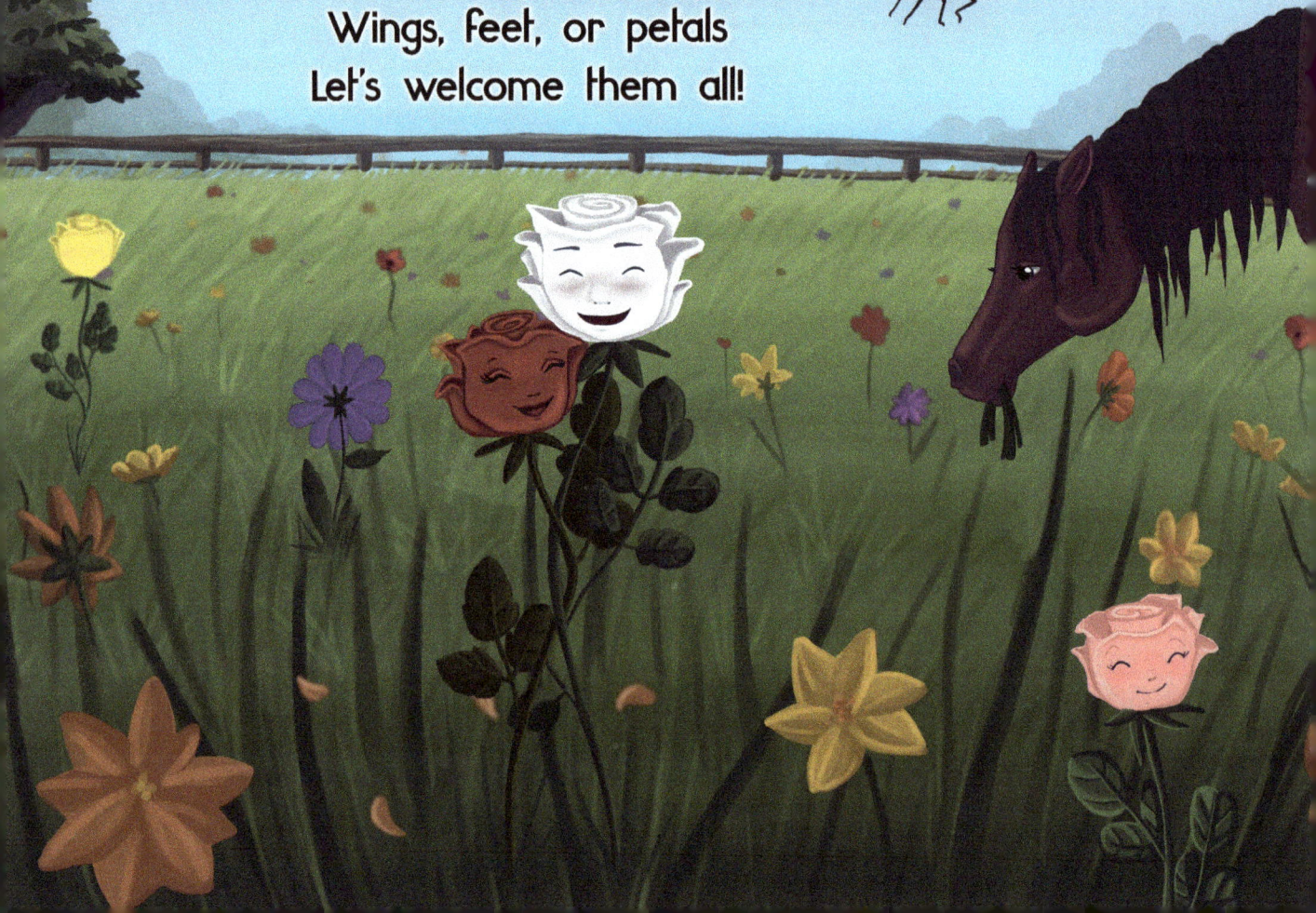

www.ingramcontent.com/pod-product-compliance
Lightning Source LLC
Chambersburg PA
CBHW041610260326
41914CB00012B/1451